Trigeminal Neuralgia

Living with trigeminal neuralgia, a practical guide.

By

Victor Venfield

Table of Contents

Introduction

Trigeminal Neuralgia is a condition in which severe facial pain affects one or both sides of the face.

It is a long term (or 'chronic') condition for which there is no cure and which may worsen over time. Sometimes an operation can provide complete pain relief.

This book has been written for people suffering from the condition. It also has advice for their families and carers on how to help someone with trigeminal neuralgia adjust to the condition.

It contains information about how a diagnosis of trigeminal neuralgia may be reached and the types of treatments which may be prescribed.

As trigeminal neuralgia affects people in different ways, you'll find information on possible 'triggers' and suggestions for ways to avoid these.

There is also a section on the day-to-day management of the condition and a list of further information sources.

Chapter 1) What is Trigeminal Neuralgia?

Trigeminal neuralgia is a disease of the nervous system and is one of the most painful of chronic (long term) medical conditions, thought to affect over one million people worldwide. It is also known as *tic doulourex.*

Trigeminal neuralgia normally results from pressure on at least one branch of the fifth cranial nerve (the trigeminal nerve), which is responsible for transmission to the brain of sensations of touch and pain from your face, teeth or mouth.

Characterized by sometimes sudden onset, severe, piercing or stabbing pain, affecting one or both sides of the face, while the pain may last only for a few seconds on each occasion, episodes of recurrent attacks may last for days, weeks or even months at a time.

Trigeminal neuralgia is more common in women than men and is most common between the ages of 60 and 70. It is rare for someone under the age of 40 years to suffer with the condition.

The pain caused by trigeminal neuralgia can make it difficult for sufferers to carry out their normal activities and some people can become isolated and susceptible to depression as a result.

An Overview

The trigeminal nerves are the largest nerves in the skull. There are two of them: one on each side of the face. Each is split into three, with each of the three branches transmitting different sensations of touch and pain back to the brain from the face, teeth or mouth.

The Trigeminal Nerve

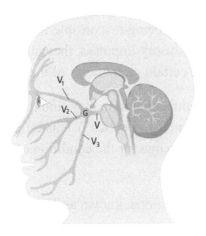

The upper branch of the nerve is the *ophthalmic* branch (V1 on diagram) which transmits sensations from the skin in the area above your eyes, your forehead and the front of your head.

The middle – *maxillary* – branch (V2 on diagram) functions along the sides of your nose, the skin on your cheeks, your upper jaw and its teeth and gums.

The third, *mandibular* branch (V3 on diagram) affects sensory perception along the lower jaw and its teeth and gums.

One, or sometimes more than one of these branches can be affected by trigeminal neuralgia, with the maxillary branch the most commonly affected and the ophthalmic branch the least commonly affected.

You will usually feel pain as a response to sensations in the area of the face served by one of the branches of the trigeminal nerve.

You may be affected on one or, more rarely, on both sides of the face.

The trigeminal nerves function both as a sensory and motor nerves. This means that, apart from being responsible for the perception, and transmission of sensory impulses, they also play an important role in controlling certain movements of the face.

Therefore, someone with trigeminal neuralgia may find they develop small involuntary movements - or 'tics.') This effect has given the condition its alternative name for the condition of *tic doloureux.*

Trigeminal neuralgia has three variations: known as Type 1, Type 2 and Symptomatic.

- In Type 1 – which is regarded as the 'classic' type – the pain caused is not constant. It is felt as a stabbing or piercing sensation. It has been likened to receiving an electric shock, and may have no identifiable cause.

- In Type 2 – also called 'atypical' – the pain is felt more constantly. It presents as a throbbing, burning or aching pain.

- Type 3 – The pain is found to be due to an underlying cause, commonly a tumor or multiple sclerosis.

The incidence of newly diagnosed cases in the United States averages approximately 4.3 per 100,000 individuals annually. *(As reported by The Facial Pain Association, 2014 Accessed June 2014.)* Figures for the UK - as reported by the NHS - are similar.

Perhaps if you read the explanation from different sources, you will understand the condition better so here is another explanation:

What is the trigeminal nerve?

The trigeminal nerve (also called the fifth cranial nerve) is one of the main nerves of the face. There is one on each side. It comes through the skull from the brain in front of the ear. It is called *tri* geminal as it splits into three main branches. Each branch divides into many smaller nerves.

The nerves from the first branch go to your scalp, forehead and around your eye. The nerves from the second branch go to the area around your cheek. The nerves from the third branch go to the area around your jaw.

The branches of the trigeminal nerve take sensations of touch and pain to the brain from your face, teeth and mouth. The trigeminal nerve also controls the muscles used in chewing and the production of saliva and tears.

Trigeminal nerve and its branches

1st branch (opthalmic)

2nd branch (maxillary)

3rd branch (mandibular)

Source: www.patients.co.uk

And another one:

Trigeminal neuralgia is caused by pain coming from your trigeminal nerve, which is also known as the fifth cranial nerve. This nerve supplies sensation to the skin on your face and the upper half of your head. It has three divisions, or branches.

- Mandibular. This runs over your lower jaw, teeth and gums.
- Maxillary. This runs through your cheek.
- Ophthalmic. This runs above your eye, forehead and the front of your scalp.

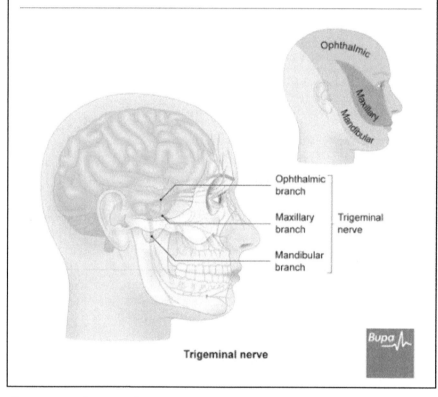

Trigeminal nerve

Source: www.bupa.co.uk

10

Chapter 2) What Causes Trigeminal Neuralgia?

There is no one definitive cause of trigeminal neuralgia. However, in up to 80-90% of cases, the condition is found to be caused by a compression of the trigeminal nerve by a blood vessel just where it enters the brain stem: the part of the brain which merges with the spinal cord.

Your trigeminal nerve is a bit like an electric cable, which has inside it lots of fibers carrying different messages to your brain. Each fiber is insulated - or protected - by a myelin sheath.

Any injury to this sheath, such as pressure from a blood vessel, can expose the nerve and causes it to misfire, sending out too many pain signals.

Sometimes, the fibers carrying the 'pain' messages touch those carrying messages about various facial stimulation, causing what amounts to a short circuit and leading to incorrect signals being sent to your brain.

This may happen in response to the slightest of stimuli, for example, mild vibration or breezes brushing the affected facial areas.

This process goes on and on in a vicious cycle, leading to the intermittent nature of the symptoms experienced by many people diagnosed with trigeminal neuralgia.

While compression of the trigeminal nerve is the most common cause of trigeminal neuralgia, others include the presence of a tumor or cyst or having multiple sclerosis (MS). (In MS, the body's immune system can attack its central nervous system, resulting in damage to nerves including the trigeminal.)

There is also a theory that suffering from shingles can cause post-herpetic neuralgia (a viral infection) and that this could be related to developing trigeminal neuralgia. Such a link has not, however, been firmly established.

Chapter 3) What Are the Symptoms of Trigeminal Neuralgia?

Symptoms

If you suffer from trigeminal neuralgia, you may find you experience pain in a variety of everyday situations such as talking to friends, eating, cleaning your teeth or shaving. (Some doctors have reported that patients have missed shaving the affected side of their face in an effort to stop the pain, or to avoid triggering a pain episode.)

Individuals with trigeminal neuralgia who suffer pain during eating, especially as they chew or swallow their food, may lose interest in eating, and a decreased food intake could lead to nutritional problems, weight loss or anorexia.

Trigeminal neuralgic pain can come on very suddenly and will last anything from a few seconds to several minutes on each occasion.

You may experience numbness or a slight tingling feeling in your face before you feel the pain. During the course of an attack, your face may feel as though it is aching or, sometimes, burning.

If you are diagnosed as suffering from typical ('Type 1'or 'classic') trigeminal neuralgia, the attacks of pain may occur regularly for a few days or weeks or months at a time, but then disappear for months or even years.

However, if you have atypical neuralgia (Type 2), then you may experience prolonged episodes of pain in between attacks. These episodes might be felt as an ache or as a burning or throbbing sensation.

In the most severe cases of trigeminal neuralgia, you may have pain episodes hundreds of times a day.

As the condition can be so unpredictable and your quality of life compromised, trigeminal neuralgia can lead to feelings of depression or despair.

Trigeminal Neuralgia and Cluster Headaches

People who suffer from cluster headaches may mistake them for trigeminal neuralgia.

While there are some similarities, there are some distinct differences too.

Cluster headaches produce a severe headache which may last for several hours. These headaches may recur in bouts lasting up to several months at a time. You may then go into remission and not experience any more for months or even years.

Often, cluster headaches will start at night and you'll find the pain is worse when you're lying down.

The pain of a cluster headache will be steady. The pain of trigeminal neuralgia has a sudden onset and is often described as like suffering an electric shock.

Unlike trigeminal neuralgia, if you are suffering from cluster headaches, you won't make the pain worse by touching your face.

Some people find that their eyes water or appear red with cluster headaches, which should not be the case with trigeminal neuralgia.

Chapter 4) How Will Trigeminal Neuralgia Affect Me?

The main problem with trigeminal neuralgia is the presence of facial pain that varies in intensity and duration. The pain usually has a sudden onset and has been described by sufferers as being like an electric shock or a feeling that their face is being crushed or is exploding, or a shooting or burning pain that cannot be relieved by medicines.

This pain is generally felt in a specific area and in response to a specific trigger, which could be a certain movement or action.

Depending on which branch of the trigeminal nerve is affected, triggers could include:

- Moving your head

- A light touch to your face

- Washing your face

- Shaving

- Applying makeup

- A cool breeze or air current (e.g. from air conditioning) felt on your face

- Smiling

- Talking

- Brushing your teeth

- Chewing

- Swallowing

Sometimes, the presence of high pitched loud noises, such as turning up the radio volume, or being in a concert hall, or on a busy street, could trigger an attack.

In some people, however, the pain may occur without specific triggers.

You may find it useful to keep a diary detailing your pain attacks: what you were doing at the time when the attack started, how it affected you, and for how long, to see if a pattern can be established.

Not only will this help you to identify your own 'triggers' but it could be helpful when discussing your condition with your physician or surgeon.

As you'll have seen from the list of potential triggers, many are everyday activities. Once you've identified what your triggers are, although you won't be able to remove them completely, you'll be able to make adjustments to minimize their effects.

Chapter 5) How is Trigeminal Neuralgia Diagnosed?

When you start getting episodes of facial pain, particularly if your gums, teeth or jaws are affected, you may first visit a dentist, (who will take a dental x-ray), rather than a physician.

While this seems logical, it may delay a diagnosis as, if your **do** have trigeminal neuralgia, the removal of, for example, a cracked tooth will not resolve the problem and the pain will persist.

It may, therefore, take some time for trigeminal neuralgia to be correctly diagnosed by going down this route. Indeed, some people spend time and money on a series of costly treatments without experiencing any pain relief before dental problems are ruled out as a cause of their pain.

If you visit your physician with symptoms of facial pain, he or she will determine which parts of your face are particularly painful by careful examination of

- your head and neck

- your mouth

- your teeth

- the joint in your lower jaw

- your ears

In order to check the involvement of the trigeminal nerve, both its motor and sensory functions may be tested.

For example, any tremors of the muscles in your face or any involuntary 'chewing' movements or spasms would show an abnormality in the function of your facial muscles.

You could be asked to open, close and move your jaw, with and without clenching your teeth. Any abnormality in the trigeminal nerve motor function could be indicated by the movement of the jaw towards the side of the face which is affected when your mouth is open.

The physician might also test the sensitivity of various areas of the face, served by different branches of the trigeminal nerve. So your reactions to being touched on the cheeks, jaw, forehead, inside your mouth or on the cornea in your eye could be recorded.

Such an examination allows the physician to discount other causes of your pain and to establish that you do have typical (or type 1) trigeminal neuralgia, rather than atypical (or type 2.)

If you have type 2, then you will not only suffer from more constant severe pain episodes, but you will also feel pain attacks – sometimes prolonged – between these episodes. Type 2 trigeminal neuralgia typically responds less well to treatment than Type 1.

If your trigeminal neuralgia **is** type 2, the focus of treatment will be the underlying condition, which could be a tumor or multiple sclerosis.

As trigeminal neuralgia is rare in people below the age of 40, if you are in this age group, your physician will certainly want to explore other causes for your facial pain.

Your physician may order an MRI (magnetic resonance imaging) scan, which will show whether your trigeminal nerve is being compressed.

Other causes of symptomatic facial pain, such as a tumor near the base of the skull or multiple sclerosis can also be investigated or discounted by the MRI scan.

What happens during an MRI Scan?

The MRI scan will use magnetic fields and radio waves to produce detailed pictures of the interior of your brain and the trigeminal nerve.

As the scanner uses very strong magnets, you will be asked whether you have

- An artificial heart valve

- A pacemaker

- Any metallic implants, for example replacement joints

- If you have had metal enter your eyes, perhaps as the result of an accident or welding work

- Whether you have had any surgery performed on your head

Before having the scan you will have to remove any jewellery, spectacles (if you wear them), metal hair slides and any dentures on a metal plate, or metal orthodontic braces.

You'll also have to leave your mobile phone, watch and bank cards outside to avoid having them damaged by the scanner.

During the scan you'll lie on a table which will move into the tunnel within the scanner.

Although staff will be able to speak to you throughout the procedure, some people do find the experience claustrophobic. If you are at all anxious, or prone to claustrophobia, discuss your concerns with the staff before the scan begins, as it is very important that you stay still during the procedure.

The scanning machine is noisy but the scan is painless and should be completed with about 45 minutes, depending on how many sets of pictures need to be taken.

Once the scan is finished, you will not feel any after effects and will be able to get on with your normal routine.

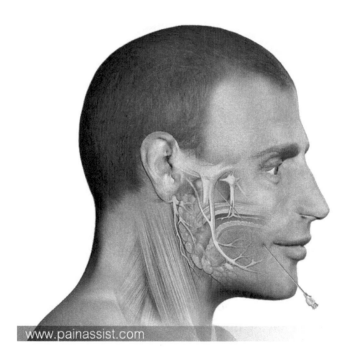

www.painassist.com

Chapter 6) How Will My Trigeminal Neuralgia Be Treated?

The first steps

As the symptoms of trigeminal neuralgia can be so debilitating and have such an effect on your everyday life, treatment should be started as soon as the condition has been diagnosed.

This should prevent your symptoms from becoming worse and potentially leading to depression and other psychosocial and physical problems.

As the most obvious effect of trigeminal neuralgia is sudden onset pain, your physician will likely prescribe painkilling medicine as soon as the condition has been diagnosed.

Painkillers such as *Paracetemol* are not effective with trigeminal neuralgic pain, but your physician may prescribe instead an anticonvulsant – such as one used to treat seizures in patients with epilepsy.

The most common anticonvulsant drug prescribed for trigeminal neuralgia is *Carbamazepine,* which is normally taken once or twice a day, though some people may need to take a higher dose from the outset.

Unfortunately, *Carbamazepine* has a number of possible side effects and some people, especially the elderly, may find it difficult to take.

Known side effects include:

- feeling nauseous

- vomiting

- tiredness

- feeling dizzy

- difficulty in controlling some movements

- a reduction in white blood cell count

- changes in the level of enzymes in your liver

- a reduction in white blood cell count

Other less common effects include:

- a dry mouth

- weight gain

- fluid retention

- headache

- blurred vision or double vision

- confusion

- problems with memory

- abnormal movement of the eyes

- uncontrollable tremors

- constipation or diarrhea

If your ethnicity is Chinese or Thai, then you may be asked to take a blood test before starting to take *Carbamazepine,* due to an ethnic vulnerability to developing a severe rash from using this medication.

There is also evidence linking the use of anticonvulsants to feelings of self-harm or even suicide.

If you are prescribed *Carbamazepine* and it proves not to be effective, or is unsuitable for you due to adverse side effects, you should ask your physician for an alternative. (*Gabapentin* is another anticonvulsant medication which may be offered.)

Other drug treatment options
Sometimes, common tricyclic anti-depressants such as *nortriptyline* or *amitriptyline* may be prescribed.

While these drugs were not developed for primarily for use with trigeminal neuralgia, they will slow down the electrical impulses resulting from the misfiring of your overactive nerve fibers, and so reduce the transmission of their pain signals and the resulting pain.

These drugs may have the added benefit of helping with the feelings of depression sometimes associated with trigeminal neuralgia.

Sometimes a drug which has been licensed for certain conditions may be found to be effective for other conditions. However, it may not have been subject to clinical trials (for safety and effectiveness) for the other conditions.

You might be offered the option of using an unlicensed treatment if your physician feels that the likely benefits seem to balance or outweigh potential risks. However, he or she should always discuss this treatment option with you before proceeding.

You might be prescribed a combination of medication as it may take some time to find a medication regime that deals adequately with your trigeminal neuralgic pain without causing too many side effects.

Referral on to a specialist
Trigeminal neuralgia is progressive so, over time, you may find that the medication you've been prescribed becomes less effective or stops working altogether, because, while it may numb the pain, it will not address the cause.

Or you may be suffering from unpleasant side effects which are compromising your quality of life, or experiencing facial pain between your spasms of trigeminal neuralgia. Or, you may simply not want to take medication indefinitely.

In such circumstances, your physician may refer you on to another healthcare specialist. This could be either:

- A pain specialist: who will assess the severity of your pain and may prescribe different or additional medication.

- A neurologist: who specializes in conditions connected to the body's central nervous system. He or she may want to carry out tests (if not already done) to rule out the presence of multiple sclerosis and, possibly, suggest changes to your medication, or

- A neurosurgeon: who, through his or her expert knowledge of the human brain and nervous system, will be able to advise on whether you might benefit from surgery.

Chapter 7) Surgical Procedures for Trigeminal Neuralgia

There are a number of neurosurgical procedures now available to treat trigeminal neuralgia. The procedure offered will depend on the nature of your pain, which part(s) of the trigeminal nerve are involved and other factors such as your general health and preference.

Some procedures are only suitable if you have classic (Type 1) trigeminal neuralgia. If you have been given an incorrect diagnosis, surgery could even make your condition worse.

While some procedures can be carried out on an outpatient basis, the more complex operations will require you to undergo general anesthesia and therefore become an inpatient.

Each procedure or operation carries its own risks, and sometimes, while the procedure may initially seem to have relieved your symptoms, they may return.

You should also be aware of the general risks associated with surgery, which – depending on the surgical procedure you have - may include hearing loss, infection, balance problems, a leak of cerebrospinal fluid and, rarely, stroke.

Occasionally people undergoing surgery for trigeminal neuralgia suffer the complication known as anesthesia dolorosa (or AD). If the trigeminal nerve is damaged during surgery, numbness may result, but you will still feel pain, despite the numbness.

This pain is often constant and may be described as burning. Further surgical procedures for someone with AD may make the condition worse.

Your surgeon should always discuss with you why he or she has recommended a particular surgery and what the risks could be, so that you can give informed consent.

a) Glycerol Injection

The procedure

In this procedure, you will be heavily sedated and your cheek will be anesthetized. The surgeon will then be able to pass a needle through your cheek, close to your mouth, and, guided by x-ray, inject glycerol into the junction of the three branches of the trigeminal nerve as it exits the skull towards your face.

This procedure should be complete within a few minutes and you should be able to go home the same day.

After effects

After this procedure, you may find that your symptoms may become slightly worse initially, particularly if you have any bruising to your cheek. You might also have pain in your jaw which can be relieved by *Paracetemol.*

Risks

- bruising and hemorrhage of your face and neck

- numbness in your face

- failure of this therapy to provide long term relief. Glycerol injection therapy may only provide temporary relief from your pain and may need to be repeated within 12 months. It can, however, be repeated many times.

You might be offered a procedure known as a rhizotomy which involves the nerve fibers been deliberately damaged in order to block pain signals. There are several different types of rhizotomy offered for trigeminal neuralgia.

b) Balloon Compression

The procedure

In this procedure a small balloon is inflated over the branch of the trigeminal nerve associated with the sensation of a light touch on your face. This relieves pressure on the nerve.

While you are under general anesthesia, the surgeon will insert a tiny tube (a cannula) through your cheek and guide it to the correct position in relation to the trigeminal nerve.

He or she will then insert a catheter with a balloon tip through the cannula. Once in position, the balloon is inflated and it squeezes part of the nerve against the brain covering. After a very short time the balloon can be deflated and will be removed, together with the catheter and the cannula.

After effects

You can normally have this procedure as an outpatient. You may remain on any medication you were taking before the procedure, before being weaned off it as directed by your surgeon.

Risks

The main risk of this procedure is of developing anesthesia dolorosa, which results in numbness to the surface of the face accompanied by a deep burning sensation. There is currently no treatment known to be effective in dealing with this.

c) Radiofrequency Thermal Lesioning

The procedure

This procedure works by injuring the endings of the nerve fibers which are causing the patient's pain.

If you are having this procedure, you will be anaesthetized and a small needle will be passed through the cheek in the same way as described for the balloon compression technique.

Once the needle is in position, you will be woken, briefly, while an electric current is passed through the needle. This will cause a slight tingling sensation in the area where the needle tip is resting.

The surgeon may then reposition the needle until the tingling is happening in the area which gives you the most trigeminal neuralgic pain.

You will then be sedated once again while the electrode heats the nerve, damaging its fibers and reducing the painful sensations you normally experience.

After effects

You can normally have this procedure as outpatient day surgery

Risks

Like the balloon compression procedure described above, this procedure carries with it the risk of developing anesthesia dolorosa, which results in numbness to the surface of the face accompanied by a deep burning sensation. There is currently no treatment known to be effective in dealing with this.

d) Stereotatic Radiosurgery (also called Gamma Knife or Cyber Knife)

The procedure

This relatively new treatment directs concentrated radiation to the point where the trigeminal nerve emerges from the brain stem. The surgeon will use computer imaging to help locate the correct position to focus the radiation on.

The effect of the radiation is to form a small lesion on the trigeminal nerve which disrupts and reduces the transmission of sensory pain signals to your brain.

For this procedure you will not need to be anaesthetized.

After effects

You may not experience any pain relief until several weeks (sometimes several months) after having this procedure.

According to figures produced by The International RadioSurgery Association, between 50% and 78% of patients treated for trigeminal neuralgia by this method report 'excellent' pain relief within a few weeks.

However, almost half of the patients treated successfully have a recurrence of pain within three years, according to www.ninds.nih.gov

Risks

- facial numbness and, (less commonly):

- loss of sense of taste

- some numbness in the eyes

- deafness

e) Microvascular Decompression (MVD)

The procedure

This is the most invasive of the possible procedures to treat trigeminal neuralgia, but it also appears to be the most effective.

For this procedure, you'll need to be an inpatient and undergo general anesthesia.

During the operation, your surgeon will make a small opening through the bone behind one of your ears. Then, he or she will move the blood vessel which is compressing your trigeminal nerve away and put a soft cushioning between it and the nerve to prevent further pressure.

If no blood vessel is shown to be pressing on the nerve, your surgeon may decide to perform a neurectomy (or partial nerve section.) This involves part of the nerve being cut close to its entrance point to the brain stem. A neurectomy can also be performed by the surgeon cutting superficial branches of the trigeminal nerve in the face.

After effects

You may need to spend some days in hospital to recuperate following this surgery and follow this with several weeks' recovery at home.

If a neurectomy has been performed during your MVD, you may experience numbness in the facial area where either the nerve or branch of the nerve has been cut.

However, the nerve may grow back and you may regain sensation in your face. A neurectomy can be performed more than once in people who suffer recurrent pain episodes.

Risks

- hearing loss

- loss of sensation in the face (often only temporary)

- meningitis

- stroke

- MVD is generally less successful for patients with type 2 trigeminal neuralgia. (

f) Botox

Some neurologists are now offering Botox injections as a means of pain control for trigeminal neuralgia. However, the relief may only be temporary and more research is needed into this treatment method.

None of the procedures described promises permanent relief from your symptoms and you should, therefore, discuss with your neurosurgeon the latest information on how soon your symptoms might recur following any particular treatment.

Chapter 8) Complementary Treatment Options for Trigeminal Neuralgia

Some people with trigeminal neuralgia find that they can manage their pain better if they use complementary therapies alongside any other medical or surgical treatment they are receiving.

Though such therapies have not been clinically proven to have any effectiveness, they may help by promoting a feeling a general wellbeing.

Before beginning any kind of complementary therapy, it is important to talk to your physician to see if there are any contraindications related to your trigeminal neuralgia.

Also, always check that the practitioner you choose is fully qualified.

A course of sessions will probably be recommended for any of the following so you should be aware that a time and financial commitment will be involved.

Acupuncture

Acupuncture has its roots in traditional Chinese medicine. Long pins or needles are inserted into the body at precise points along the body's meridians (pathways) in order to block pain signals, reducing the intensity of the patient's pain.

It is very important to use an acupuncturist who is well trained and qualified, as permanent nerve damage could result from consulting an unqualified practitioner. Always ask to see certificates if none are displayed.

Acupuncture treatment for trigeminal neuralgia would involve the insertion of single-use, disposable needles along the path of the nerve and its branches along whichever side of your face is affected.

You might feel a slight discomfort as the needles are inserted and may remain conscious of them during treatment, but this is something you should become used to if you have a course of treatments.

Once the needles have been correctly positioned, you will be asked to relax. Many patients find acupuncture promotes deep relaxation. The acupuncturist may manipulate the needles while they are in situ.

The length of time the needles are left in position will vary. In many cases, some pain relief is felt right away but further or regular treatments may be suggested.

Accupressure

Less invasive than acupuncture, acupressure works on a similar principle but with the application of pressure, rather than the insertion of needles, to the meridians. It may therefore be a better option for anyone who has tried acupuncture but found it too uncomfortable, or who has a fear of needles.

As with acupuncture, you should only consult a qualified and experienced practitioner.

Chiropractic

In chiropractic medicine, treatment is concentrated on identifying and correcting subtle alignment problems in the patient's spine.

As the trigeminal nerves exit the base of the skull, the portion of the spine closest to the skull may be the focus of treatment work, as it thought that misalignment in this area can cause pressure to the trigeminal nerve.

Before chiropractic treatment, an x-ray will usually be taken so that the chiropractor can see both the area to be worked on and the degree of adjustment needed.

Treatment may be needed on a very regular basis to begin with and then periodically to check that any improvement is being maintained.

According to TNA The Facial Pain Association in the US, good results have been obtained from a sub field of chiropractic known as UCC which concentrates on the alignment of the atlas (the top vertebrae in your spine.) However, as yet, only a small proportion of chiropractors offer this specific treatment option.

Reflexology

In reflexology, massage is applied to various points on the feet, hands, legs and parts of the head, (called reflex points), which are believed to correspond to certain body parts.

By targeting the point corresponding to the trigeminal nerve, the practitioner may be able to offer pain relief.

Meditation

Meditation is used by many people as a way of relaxing and calming the mind and creating a sense of inner peace. It can also be used to help in pain relief, either in conjunction with conventional medical or surgical treatments or, for some people, as a preferred therapy which does not rely on drugs or surgery.

Mindfulness is a form of meditation which could be helpful for trigeminal neuralgia sufferers as it teaches you to concentrate on the present moment and learn to accept and relax into the pain and so manage it better.

With regular practice, people who meditate may also find that it helps them deal with feelings of depression and increase their sense of general wellbeing.

(Details of peoples' experiences of using meditation to help deal with trigeminal neuralgia can be found through various forums and blogs, details of which are listed in chapter 12.)

Tai chi

Based on a sequence of gentle movements between specific postures and linked to the pattern of your breathing, tai chi may be helpful in promoting wellbeing and a feeling of calm, which could be used to distract from, and reduce the pain of, trigeminal neuralgia.

Search the internet or your local paper for details of classes in your area. Make sure that your instructor is qualified and that he or she knows about your condition.

Yoga

Like tai chi, the potential benefits of yoga for trigeminal neuralgia sufferers lie in the concentration needed to achieve the postures, which may offer helpful distraction from painful symptoms, while also promoting a general feeling of wellbeing.

There are many different types of yoga now widely on offer and you may need to try out a few different types before settling on one that suits you.

Mention your condition to your teacher who should be able to advise on any postures to avoid, or adapt postures to suit you.

Search the internet or your local paper for details of classes in your area.

Biofeedback

Actions such as clapping our hands, waving to a friend, kicking and winking are actions that we can control. The rest of our bodily functions - such as blood pressure, heart rate and body temperature - are involuntary actions or responses to our environment.

Biofeedback is a technique used to help us gain more control over the involuntary mechanisms in our body. There are different types of biofeedback, but one commonly used with patients who have trigeminal neuralgia is neurofeedback using an EEG.

During a biofeedback session, electrodes are attached to the skin and send signals to a monitor to highlight involuntary movements. This helps the physician and patient focus on the effects of making small, subtle changes in movements, e.g. relaxing muscles, which could help relieve pain.

Repeated sessions will be needed to 'train' your body to deal with involuntary pain signals.

Homeopathy

While there is, as yet, no definitive homeopathic remedy for trigeminal neuralgia, if you are interested in using homeopathy, you may find a practitioner who will offer suggestions for treating you in a holistic way, with the aim of helping your body to deal with the underlying causes of the condition and the painful symptoms associated with an attack.

Ayurvedic medicine

Ayurveda originated in India and seeks to maintain the balance between body, mind and spirit through natural medication, diet, oils and massage, individually or in combination.

If you can't find a practitioner, there are numerous books available about this practice.

Chapter 9) Living with Trigeminal Neuralgia

Being diagnosed with trigeminal neuralgia can present many challenges. The pain may be constant or episodic but it is often debilitating, making everyday activities difficult.

In addition, medication, and even surgery, may not offer long term relief and sufferers can become liable to feelings of depression, leading to social isolation.

As trigeminal neuralgia affects different people in different ways, according to which branch of the trigeminal nerve is being constricted, not everyone's pain will be triggered in the same way.

However, you will get to know what your own triggers are and you can begin to make small adjustments to your routines to help minimize your pain.

Some suggestions are given below. You will also find lots of further suggestions from other TM sufferers on the internet via various blogs. See chapter 12.

Avoid touching your face and having it touched

- Try and minimize kissing and hugging when greeting people, as stimulation of the face could increase your pain.

- When using the phone, use the speakerphone setting so that you don't have to press the receiver to your face.

Avoid extremes of cold

- Keep as much of your face as possible covered with a scarf when outdoors during cold or breezy weather.

- Avoid sitting close to an open window or even being in a draft, whether from a window or air conditioning unit. Keep your car window closed as much as possible.

Apply heat

- Some people have found that actively applying heat – such as a heated beanbag or pad – to the painful area of the face seems to relax the nerve and relieve their pain.

- Keep some disposable instant warm packs with you in case you suddenly feel a chill. You'll find it more comfortable apply the heated pack through a scarf, rather than directly onto your face.

- Using a heat pad can also help to relax the muscles in your neck and help you if you're finding sleep difficult due to the pain.

Modify your mealtime routines

- If your trigeminal neuralgia is affecting the lower (mandibular) branch of the nerve, you may experience pain in your teeth, gums and lower jaw, which can impact when you are trying to eat or drink.

- Try taking smaller mouthfuls than you would normally, to minimize the amount of facial movement needed.

- If you find chewing is a particular trigger, have a good supply of soft foods available to substitute in meals, or make alternative choices, such as mashed potato instead of fries.

- Because a damaged trigeminal nerve has increased sensitivity to stimuli, avoid eating or drinking anything which is either very cold or very hot to prevent triggering a pain episode.

- Wait till a hot drink has cooled to room temperature and avoid ice in cold drinks. (You can use a straw to help stop a drink being in contact with the most painful areas of your mouth.)

- As caffeine is a nerve stimulant, you may want to consider limiting your intake.

- You may not feel like cooking when you are having an attack but eating easily available 'junk' food may simply make things worse.

- Instead, try and have some healthy options ready prepared and frozen, which you can use during an attack.

- You may not feel much like eating but try and keep to a regular routine of meals. If you have severe pain, you may find it helpful to take smaller, more frequent meals so that your facial muscles have less work to do at each meal and have time to rest between meals.

- Make time to eat in a quiet and relaxed atmosphere. Don't rush a meal because you're supposed to be somewhere else.

- If you find that eating or drinking are major trigger factors for your trigeminal neuralgia, discuss this with your physician who may be able to refer you to a dietician. You can then be sure that, despite any adjustments you make to your diet, you will still be getting all the right nutrients.

Lifestyle changes

As trigeminal neuralgia is thought to be caused by pressure from a blood vessel on the affected trigeminal nerve and its branches, it makes sense to minimize activities such as smoking which over time can put pressure on your blood vessels and impede circulation.

Cutting down on smoking and drinking may help to decrease the amount of pain attacks and their severity.

Modify your daily routines

As well as altering your eating and/or drinking habits, you may find that you can modify other daily activities in order to minimize the physical and emotional impact of your trigeminal neuralgia.

For example, instead of rubbing your face between your hands when washing, you could lightly touch a warm cloth to your face instead.

Or, if you find brushing your teeth particularly painful, talk to your dentist about using a mouth rinse instead of toothpaste and a brush at times when you are having a pain attack.

Supplements

Some trigeminal neuralgia patients have found taking supplements containing B vitamins or taking multivitamins, Omega 3 fish oil or magnesium to be helpful.

You will find many websites where sufferers share tips. However, it is always advisable to check with your physician before taking supplements.

Exercise

Suffering with trigeminal neuralgia doesn't mean that you can't exercise. Indeed many sufferers find that doing the type of exercise they most enjoy can help them cope with the symptoms, even if they are having a mild pain attack at the time.

It would be worth checking with your physician first before taking up any new kind of exercise.

Visiting your dentist

You may be anxious about visiting your dentist generally but may feel even more concerned about pain when you have trigeminal neuralgia.

TNA The Facial Pain Association has some useful tips on how to manage your dental consultation at: www.fpa-support.org including trying to time your appointment to avoid a pain episode. If you let your dentist know that you have trigeminal neuralgia (and this should be added to your notes), he or she may be willing to see you at short notice.

Your dentist might also suggest increasing your dose of medication for a few days before the treatment and also afterwards.

If you can indicate the most sensitive areas to your dentist, he or she should be able to treat those areas last and offer a topical numbing treatment if needed.

Whilst you may be anxious about your dental treatment, if you discuss any concerns beforehand, you will find that your dentist will be sympathetic and will try to adjust the way he or she works to give you the best possible experience and it is, of course, important that you continue to care for your teeth despite your trigeminal neuralgia.

Know your limits

You will almost inevitably have to make some changes to your normal routines to accommodate your trigeminal neuralgia.

Make sure that you give yourself plenty of leeway and flexibility with times, deadlines etc. so that you do not feel that pressured or anxious. Recognise and know your own triggers and limitations and be kind to yourself. A positive attitude will allow you to cope better with the disease.

Chapter 10) Caring For Someone Who Has Trigeminal Neuralgia

Living with, or have caring responsibilities for, someone who has trigeminal neuralgia can be challenging.

The unpredictability of the condition means that the sufferer will not usually have advance warning of a pain attack. Attacks may be several days or weeks apart, or could occur as frequently as several hundred times a day.

It is important to find out as much as you can about the condition generally, and how it affects the person you care for specifically, from them and their doctor or surgeon (with the person's permission). You will also find information and support from other carers on various websites. See chapter 12 for details.

A calm, sympathetic and patient approach to the person's pain attacks and any associated anxiety or depression will be much appreciated.

Signs of an attack

While they are having a pain attack, you may notice that the person's face twitches involuntarily or they may reach towards the painful area (though actually touching it could increase the pain.) They may also cry out in pain.

If the person has suffered with trigeminal neuralgia for some time, they should be able to identify situations which could trigger an attack (for example, sitting near an open window or having a car window open) and will avoid these where possible.

You should aim to help them find ways of avoiding trigger situations and, perhaps, modify their daily routine, so that they can live as normal a life as possible.

Mealtimes

If someone's trigeminal neuralgia is particularly affecting their jaws, teeth or gums, this can have a significant impact at mealtimes.

- They may seem hesitant about eating, or eat very slowly, fearful of triggering an attack.

- They might be reluctant to eat with other people in social situations in case they suffer an attack.

You should be watchful for any problems and, if you are in company, you could contribute more to the conversation to give the person some time to recover.

You might need to help them adjust their schedule of meals, offering smaller amounts of food more frequently.

Effects of medication

There are a range of drugs used to treat trigeminal neuralgia including anticonvulsant medications. These work by suppressing the pain signals between the brain and the part of the face affected by trigeminal neuralgia.

If the person you care for is taking a high dose of anticonvulsant medication, they could be subject to confusion, or have difficulty in retaining information or recalling words. If this happens, you should record specific instances and talk to the person's physician (or remind them to mention it to the physician), as an alternative drug might be available.

Try and be sensitive when reminding someone of a forgotten word or date, so that they will not feel embarrassed.

Some medication may also cause fatigue and drowsiness which can impact on the person's daily routine as their energy levels fluctuate. Again, sensitivity and a willingness to adapt routine will be appreciated.

Mental health

People who suffer from trigeminal neuralgia can be subject to depression or, in extreme cases, suicidal thoughts.

Someone who has recently begun to suffer from the condition may find the process of diagnosis difficult and dispiriting to deal with.

If they have had the condition for some time, they may have been through several drug regimes and surgery, without long term relief.

Unfortunately trigeminal neuralgia is classed as a chronic condition, for which there is no cure.

As a carer, you can help by being as understanding and sympathetic as possible. Let the person talk about how the condition is affecting them and their feelings about it, as and when they want to.

If they become severely depressed, formal psychiatric assessment and support may be needed, which their medical practitioner should be able to arrange.

Support groups

It is thought that 150,000 people are diagnosed with trigeminal neuralgia each year. (According to The American Association of Neurological Surgeons, 2012.)

The person you care for may find it easier to talk about their trigeminal neuralgia with others who are having similar experiences.

This 'talking' could be face-to-face or, increasingly, online, where are support groups offering help to both sufferers and their carers and families. For more details see chapter 12.

Your own health

Having caring responsibilities for someone with any kind of chronic condition is extremely tiring. For the sake of your own physical and mental wellbeing it is important that you:

- eat well

- get enough sleep

- make some time for your own social life and interests

- arrange to take occasional breaks away to 'recharge your batteries.'

Chapter 11) Developments in Understanding Trigeminal Neuralgia

Beginnings of a diagnosis

Trigeminal neuralgia (TN) is not a new disease.

What is thought to be the first description of TN is by Aretaeus, an ancient Greek physician, living in Cappadocia (now an area of Turkey), during the first century AD. He referred to a pain *'involving spasm and distortion of the countenance.'*

In the 11th century AD, Jujani, an Arab physician describes a condition involving *'unilateral face pain causing spasms and anxiety.'* He suggested that the cause of this pain might be the proximity of an artery to a nerve.

The first detailed account of the condition was written by Englishman John Fothergill who, in 1773, presented a paper to the Medical Society of London mentioning many of the features which are now associated with the condition. He also observed that it was more common in females and in older patients.

Trigeminal neuralgia is sometimes known as Fothergill's Disease but the more common alternative name – tic douloureux – was coined by Frenchman Nicolas André who believed that the

"pain originated from compression of facial sensory peripheral nerves..... he reproduced the tic pain and treated it by using careful efforts to remove adhesions from the nerve with a caustic solution of mercury water. Believing that recurrence of the pain was a result of early closure of the wound, with recompression

of the nerve being the direct cause, André prevented
recompression by ensuring open wound drainage."
(http://www.ncbi.nlm.nih.gov/pubmed/10223470MID, accessed July 2014)

Pujol, Chapman and Tiffany, working in the late 18th and 19th centuries, gave a more complete clinical picture of TN and also established ways of differentiating TN from other facial pain, for example, toothache.

The twentieth century

By the middle of the second decade of the century, modern neurosurgical treatment was being developed, and in 1932 an American, Walter Dandy, suggested that trigeminal nerve pain was most likely due to compression of a blood vessel by the trigeminal nerve.

The invasive surgical technique known as microvascular decompression (MVD) was developed throughout the 1950s and 1960s.

Now, in the 21st century, surgeons and research scientists work to achieve a balance between pain relief and the risks of neural surgery as well as investigating the potential of new techniques.

Research

Research into new treatments and techniques for trigeminal neuralgia is taking place all the time all over the world.

TNA The Facial Pain Association reported in autumn 2009 the potential use of stem cell and gene therapies for the treatment of trigeminal neuralgia.
(http://www.fpasupport.org/documents/TNAlertFall09.pdf Accessed July *2014*)

This could be by using stem cells to 'patch' or repair damaged parts of the myelin sheath around the trigeminal nerve.

Genes found to be involved in pain control could be used to replace defective genes or introduced to stimulate the growth of cells implicated in pain control.

Women are more likely to suffer from trigeminal neuralgia than men and researchers, including at the National Institute of Neurological Disorders and Stroke, are carrying out research to find out whether the female hormone estrogen may be involved in nerve pain.

This could lead to the development of medication limiting the action of estrogen on nerves and, therefore, the transmission of pain signals.

The use of using electrical stimulation to activate the body's natural opiates is being investigated at the University of Michigan. It is hoped that development of this technique could reduce a patient's need for painkillers and be more effective in pain control.

Clinical trials

If you're interested in taking part in clinical trials for potential new trigeminal neuralgia treatments, you can find more information on these websites:

If you're in the UK (correct as at July 2014):

http://www.ukctg.nihr.ac.uk

In the US, (correct as at July 2014):

http://clinicaltrials.gov

Chapter 12) Self Help Information

Insurance Cover and Financial Assistance

Most health care insurance plans and companies cover the treatment costs associated with trigeminal neuralgia. However, this may be full or partial, depending on the premiums paid and limited to the more recognized treatment regimens, such as the use of drugs and surgery.

It is, therefore, important to confirm with your health care insurance provider the extent of your cover before considering any treatments, if you are relying on health insurance to cover the cost.

In the United States, Federal and State health departments may offer assistance to those who suffer with trigeminal neuralgia under the Medicaid program. This is usually given to individuals who were considered to be indigents and cannot afford any of the treatment options.

Also, some people may qualify for disability payments because of a diagnosis of trigeminal neuralgia.

If you are in the UK, you should see your General Practitioner who may refer you for tests, scans or assessment by a surgeon. These costs should be covered by the NHS.

The cost of medication may also be met in the UK if you meet the current criteria for receiving free prescriptions.

Some surgical procedures for trigeminal neuralgia may be covered by private medical insurance in the U.K.

Support and Advice Groups

A quick internet search for *"Trigeminal Neuralgia"* shows listings for many organisations and support groups as well as blogs.

They contain information on the condition and details of support groups for people who suffer from trigeminal neuralgia and their families, with advice on how people manage their condition (including advice on therapies or supplements to try), and the latest research findings.

Details of a selection are given here:

 TNA The Facial Pain Association has general information about the condition and the various treatments available and offers an online support network and, if you register with the site, you can join in with blogs and chat to, and swap experiences with, other people who have the condition.

http://www.fpa-support.org/

The Trigeminal Neuralgia Association UK. As well as having useful free information, if you join the organisation (£15 as at July 2014), you will receive a selection of booklets with information about the condition, the various treatment options, how to cope with the pain and how to care for someone with trigeminal neuralgia.

www.*TNA.org.uk*

Patient.co.uk is an independent health site containing general information and a patient forum on trigeminal neuralgia.

http://www.patient.co.uk

Living with TN is a US based support group that aims to help individuals with trigeminal neuralgia and their families to adjust to, and live with, their condition. It offers information and forum discussions with other sufferers including details of alternative therapies and their results.

http://www.livingwithtn.org

MD Junction is US based and has a support group for trigeminal neuralgia sufferers with discussions on treatments and tips on living with the condition.

http://www.mdjunction.com

Carers UK offers advice to people caring for patients will all kinds of chronic conditions. It also has up to date information on the financial and practical support available to carers in the UK.

http://www.carersuk.org/

Social Media

There are also several Facebook groups dedicated to trigeminal neuralgia including:

https://www.facebook.com

(October 7th has been designated International Awareness Day for Trigeminal Neuralgia and Facial Pain Disorders.)

You will find posts relating to trigeminal neuralgia on Twitter.

Books

Striking Back - The Trigeminal Neuralgia and Face Pain Handbook - *a layman's guide to understanding and treating what is often called the world's worst pain*

The authors are George Weigel, an American journalist and TN patient and Dr Kenneth Casey, a neurosurgeon who has worked with Dr Peter Jannetta, the pioneer of the microvascular decompression (MVD) procedure.

This book contains information about trigeminal neuralgia and other types of facial pain, written in a way that it accessible to readers with or without a medical background and could help sufferers to make more informed choices about their treatment and care.

Insights—Facts and Stories Behind Trigeminal Neuralgia

Written by Professor Joanna Zakrzewska, a lead consultant in Facial Pain at Eastman Dental Hospital in London and international expert on trigeminal neuralgia.

The book details both patients' experiences and scientific data, from diagnosis to the best available treatments. Practical tips on coping with recurrent pain are also included and the book is a useful reference source not only for sufferers, but also for their carers and families.

Chapter 13) Conclusion

While a diagnosis of trigeminal neuralgia may be daunting, with some research, maintaining good relationships with your physician (and surgeon, if applicable) and the support or your family and friends, you should be able to find ways to manage it and reduce its impact on your life.

Here are some key points to remember:

1. If you are experiencing facial pain and have consulted a dentist, without having long term relief, you should visit your physician in case your pain is due to trigeminal neuralgia.

2. Once you realise you are having frequent episodes of facial pain, you should try and record dates and duration, together with notes about what you were doing at the time. This will be useful both to you in identifying your personal triggers and to your physician.

3. Triggers could include:

- Feeling a cold breeze on your face

- Moving your head

- A light touch to your face

- Washing your face

- Shaving

- Putting on makeup

- Smiling

- Talking

- Brushing your teeth

- Chewing

- Swallowing

- High pitched loud noises

4. By identifying your own triggers, you should be able to make lifestyle changes to help you to adjust to trigeminal neuralgia and reduce the frequency of painful attacks.

5. There is a range of treatments for trigeminal neuralgia. You will probably initially be offered medication but you may also be referred to a neurologist or neurosurgeon and have an MRI examination.

   It is important that you discuss any proposed treatments and potential side effects before giving your consent.

6. If you are going to be relying on private health insurance to pay for any treatment, you should get a quotation and discuss what is, and what is not, covered before going ahead.

7. Some trigeminal neuralgia sufferers have found alternative therapies such as acupuncture or chiropractic to be effective.

   If you are thinking of trying one of these treatments, discuss it with your physician first and always find a suitably qualified and experienced therapist. Be sure to make them aware of your diagnosis.

8. Sharing your experiences of trigeminal neuralgia with other sufferers might be helpful. You could either 'advertise' locally via your local paper or join one of the internet or social media forums dedicated to the condition.

9. You should involve your partner, family and friends in the management of your condition as far as you feel comfortable. Their support could be vital in helping you keep positive.

Sources

The following sources were consulted in the writing of this book:

http://www.nhs.uk/conditions

http://www.tna.org.uk

http://www.tna.org.uk

http://www.fpa-support.org

http://facepainhelp.com

http://www.brainandspine.org.uk

http://www.ninds.nih.gov

http://www.irjponline.com

http://www.patient.co.uk

http://www.ncbi.nlm.nih.gov

http://www.uhb.nhs.uk

http://www.kumc.edu

Published by IMB Publishing 2014

CPSIA information can be obtained at www.ICGtesting.com
Printed in the USA
LVOW01s0759150815

450252LV00031B/1323/P

9 781910 410196